VISI

AND

SCHOOL

SUCCESS

A GUIDE TO UNDERSTANDING VISION'S ROLE IN LEARNING AND WHAT THE TEACHER CAN DO TO FACILITATE LEARNING IN THE CLASSROOM.

George B. Spache, Ph.D.

Lillian R. Hinds, Ph.D.

Lois B. Bing, A.B., O.D.

VISION EXTENSION

Copyright © 1992 George B. Spache, Ph.D., Lillian R. Hinds, Ph.D., and Lois B. Bing, A.B., O.D.

Printed in the United States of America

Published by VisionExtension, Inc.
2912 South Daimler Street
Santa Ana, CA 92705-5811

Library of Congress Cataloging-in-Publication Data
    Spache, George Daniel, 1909-
        Vision and school success : a guide to understanding vision's
    role in learning in the classroom / George D. Spache, Lillian R. Hinds,
    Lois B. Bing.
        p.   cm.
        Originally published: Cleveland : Clarion, c1990.
        ISBN 0-929780-05-1.
        1. Visually handicapped children--Education. I. Hinds, Lillian R.
    II. Bing, Lois B. III. Title.
    HV1638.S63 1992
    371.91'1--dc20   92-22854
                                     CIP

TABLE OF CONTENTS

PREFACE

The relationship of children's visual defects to their academic achievement is virtually ignored by America's schools. The test widely used (the Snellen Chart) gives no real indication of the visual needs of most children. In fact, the children who fail the test are most likely to succeed in their academic efforts if they have no other major defects not measured by that test.

Here, we are trying to convey a broader concept of vision, including its sensory, motor and central processing dimensions. Research has changed the working concept of vision from being like a camera to being more like an elaborate computer system. Researchers are now saying that a third of the cortex is involved in vision processing. This manual is written to acquaint those involved in children's learning with these changes in understanding vision as it operates when learning takes place by means of seeing. Vision is considered a dynamic, complex process with central and peripheral elements. Since it is the classroom teacher who meets the student on a daily basis, it is she who must have the necessary information. We hope to help educators recognize the visual demands of the classroom, the behavior of students who are experiencing stress because of their vision problems, and ways and means of alleviating this stress.

George D. Spache, Ph.D.

I.

VISION AS IT OPERATES FOR LEARNING—THE TOTAL PROCESS INVOLVED

Vision is a Highly Complex Process

When vision is considered in relation to the ability to achieve or perform adequately, the total process of vision involved in the act must be appraised, not just a portion of it. The classical discussion of vision uses a camera to illustrate vision. This might be helpful in some respects, but this analogy might actually be a major stumbling block in understanding the total process of vision and how it operates when a child reads or learns through means of his vision. If the eye is likened to a camera, we must take cognizance of the fact that children have two eyes, so two "cameras" are involved. Sometimes the two eyes are nearly alike, and then again they can be quite different--one receiving a clear picture, while the other receives an altogether different impression of varying degrees of indistinctiveness or even of different size. Sometimes both will receive a clear picture when the object of regard is near at hand but not when it is farther away. Or one eye might receive a clear picture and the other none at all.

The Eye-Aiming Mechanisms

The process of vision differs from a camera in other important respects. Without moving at all, a camera can, in the twinkle of an eye, snap a picture of a whole page of print that is clear from top to bottom and from edge to edge. On the other hand, the eyes can see clearly only that part of the page of print which is fixated directly. The parts of the page that are off to the side are seen indistinctly. Hence, in reading a line of print it is necessary to aim the eyes at a succession of points along the line. This periodic re-aiming of the eyes is accomplished through the coordinated activity of 12 muscles, six on the outside of each eye. These muscles pull the eyes in or out, and up or down, and also twist each eye in a clockwise or counterclockwise direction around its line of sight. A highly coordinated process is involved which must function with precision to aim the two eyes at a common point and to change to another common point of fixation easily and with accuracy.

The Eye-Focusing Mechanism

We are familiar with the idea that some cameras must be focused for objects at one distance and then must be refocused in order to photograph objects at a different distance. Here again, however, the process of vision is much more involved than a camera. Focusing of the eyes is accomplished through the action of muscles within the eyes, but the focusing of the two eyes is tied together in such a way that one eye cannot change focus unless the other also changes focus. Hence, even though each eye by itself can focus on either far or near objects, the two eyes, taken together as they function in the process of vision, may fail to focus at the same distance. Lenses may have to be worn in these cases to bring the eyes into balance.

The Fusion Mechanism

The eyes constitute only the first part of the process of vision. In reading, for instance, the image of the printed words formed on the retina of each eye has to be transferred to the brain before this impression can be interpreted. The light pattern focused on the light-sensitive layer at the back of each eye (the retina) generates nerve impulses which are transmitted by way of nerve fibers to a certain portion of the surface of the brain called the visual cortex. The images from the two eyes are formed on the same surface in much the same way that identical images could be projected on the same screen with two projectors. In order to make the images coincide, the two eyes must first of all be aimed, or fixated, at a common point. The mechanism which aims and keeps the eyes properly pointed after they have changed fixation from one target to another is only one phase of fusion. The second phase of fusion is the integration of images from the two eyes into a single image.

Central Processing—Perception

In the process of vision, the integrated image from the two eyes is interpreted as an array of perceived images which lie in different directions and at different distances. They are the counterparts of the objects that lie in front of the observer. These perceived images are modified by memory from past experiences involving other sense modalities as well as vision.

The complexity of the total process of vision is increased by the interrelatedness between eye-aiming, eye-focusing, fusing the impressions from the two eyes and projecting images in the right directions and to the right distances. The whole system is actually good enough so that the observer makes no distinction between his visual images and the real objects in the physical world that produces them. This is the complex process of vision through which a child receives most of the knowledge he gains in school and in the world about him.

The Importance of Binocular (Two-Eyed) Vision

Difficulty in using the two eyes together will usually interfere with learning. Fortunately, however, this difficulty can be overcome in most cases by visual training in binocular use of the eyes under qualified professional supervision and/or by the use of special lenses.

Binocular vision has these advantages over monocular (one-eyed) vision:

1. A wider field of vision is afforded.
2. There is a better chance of seeing things at the threshold of visibility.
3. Stereopsis (the most important factor in three dimensional seeing) is possible only through binocular vision. Stereopsis is the ability to see that things have width, length and thickness or depth.
4. It provides a more precise judgment of direction and the distance of objects from the viewer.
5. From a cosmetic standpoint the child is greatly benefited.

Without binocular vision, the child tends to read with only one eye, or to alternate from one eye to the other. As a consequence, he tends to lose or omit many words and thus to lose comprehension.

Summary: Vision as it Operates for Learning

Vision, as it operates for learning, involves much more than the ability to see. The process of vision is quite complex. For study and testing purposes, we can divide vision into three general areas which are interrelated, each affecting the other. These general areas are: Sensory--sensory input from the retina transmitted along the optic nerve fibers; Motor--the control of focus, pupil size, and the direction in which the eyes are pointed, having the two eyes pointed at the same object of interest; Central Processing--the joining of the vision input and the input of the other sensory systems and their memory traces and relating these to time and space to produce the final product we call perception. Attention to what is being seen is also involved. We depict them here as: A, Sensory; B, Motor; and C, Central Processing; with D--the final perception of what is seen. A and B affect each other and control the quality of the vision input. C is highly individual, affected by the functioning of the other sensory systems and opportunities to relate what is seen with what is experienced through these other sensory systems. All three areas--Sensory, Motor and Central Processing--have to be accounted for in appraising vision as it relates to learning. The end product "D" is in turn affected also by health, nutrition, fatigue, emotion, etc. which vary from individual to individual.

II.

ELEMENTS OF THE TOTAL PROCESS OF VISION

Sensory

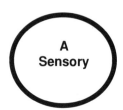

Sensory includes:

a. The structures of the eye and the nerve pathways connecting the eye with the cortex, the intactness and health state of these structures.

b. The eye as an optical instrument and its ability to produce a sharp focus on the retina (visual acuity).

Motor Mechanisms

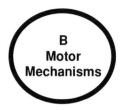

The Motor Mechanisms involve:

a. Cortical control of:

   1. Eye movements: following (pursuit), and changing fixation from one object to another (saccadic).

   2. Eye movements to integrate (fuse) into a single com-

posite image the inputs into the cortex from the two eyes.

3. The focus mechanism which changes the power of the lens within the eye to obtain a clear image at different distances. The focus mechanism is also tied into eye movements. As the focus mechanism functions, the eyes automatically receive a stimulus to converge or diverge. This stimulus for the eyes to converge or diverge is usually too weak or too strong, and fusional movements are needed to achieve a single image.

b. Peripheral structures:

1. The six muscles outside each eye that move the eye.

2. The ciliary muscle within the eye, controlling the thickness of the lens of the eye (focusing power).

Central Processing

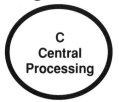

C
Central
Processing

In central processing, the vision input, after it is fused into a single composite image, is modified by past memory traces of previous vision inputs and the inputs of the other sensory systems and the past memory traces of these systems:

a. Seeing and balance.

b. Seeing and touching.

c. Seeing and hearing and naming.

d. Seeing to move and seeing to guide hands.

e. Seeing and taste, smell, hot/cold.

From the coordinated inputs of all these sensory systems these skills are developed:

a. Seeing and perceiving detail.

b. Seeing and determining position and distance of object in

7

space.
c. Seeing and labeling or naming.
d. Seeing and developing visual memory and visualization.
e. Seeing and manipulating objects.
f. Seeing and moving: hands, feet position in space.

It is in central processing that the vision input is clothed with meaning and color and projected out into space in different directions and distances.

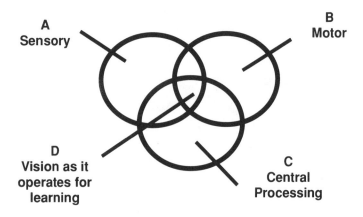

These three areas--A, Sensory; B, Motor; and C, Central Processing--act together as a unit to produce the final product D, which we call vision.

No one area can be omitted. All act together as a unit, each affecting the other. No one area can be omitted if a complete evaluation of the total process of vision is to be obtained.

III.

IMPROVING ABILITIES IN THE TOTAL PROCESS OF VISION

Sensory

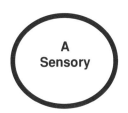

Problems and poor performance in the sensory area are alleviated or compensated for by:

a. Glasses to compensate for refractive error (farsightedness [hyperopia], nearsightedness [myopia], astigmatism [more refractive error in one area of the eye than the other], anisometropia [refractive error significantly greater in one eye than the other]) and to improve visual acuity.

b. Surgery to help a given eye see better or to help the two eyes to work together--in some cases it is done for cosmetic reasons.

c. Medication to treat pathology (pathology-anatomical deviation from normal or disease of the eye).

d. Therapy to improve visual acuity when an eye is amblyopic (amblyopic--dimness of vision not caused by refractive error or disease).

e. Therapy to improve low vision or to select low vision aids.

Treatment in the sensory area differs from that in the motor area. In the sensory area, treatment involves glasses to see clearly, medication and surgery to treat pathology, and vision training to improve visual acuity in amblyopic eyes.

Some problems due to refractive error in this area can often be detected by the usual Snellen Chart testing for visual acuity. Some problems of pathology may be observed--i.e., an eye that turns, red eyes, encrusted eyelids, or complaints of pain.

In many research reports the ability to see clearly at the distance the Snellen test is administered (20 feet) has shown little or no relationship to school achievement. It does not measure anything at reading distance and hence gives no information relevant to the child's problems at his desk.

Motor Mechanisms

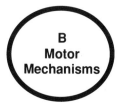

Some problems in the motor mechanisms can be detected by some of the extended vision screening programs such as the Keystone or the Titmus. However, some important abilities are not included even in these.

Treatment in this area involves:
a. Glasses to:
   1. Aid focus ability.
   2. Improve the ability to maintain single vision. Sometimes such glasses are prescribed as bifocals when lenses that are different from that needed for seeing clearly at distance are indicated when using the eyes at book and desk distances.
b. Training to improve:
   1. Pursuit (following) and saccadic (change of fixation)

eye movements.
2. The ability to obtain and maintain single vision.
3. Focus facility.

Treatment has been found to alleviate the symptoms of vision difficulty associated with the functioning of the motor mechanisms.

Central Processing

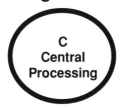

Several professions test performance in this area. A few provide some therapy.

Therapy in this area may involve interrelations between vision and the other sensory systems.
  a. Seeing and balance and orientating in space.
  b. Seeing--haptic system (related to or based on the sense of touch).
      tactual
      kinesthetic
      deep pressure
      pain
      thermal (heat or cold)
  c. Seeing--smell
      taste
  d. Seeing--hearing and speaking

All of these sensory systems affect how we perceive objects. Training through normal daily activities in this area begins at birth and continues throughout life. Some, for one reason or another, need more experiences (activities involving vision with these other sensory systems) than they have had. Significant improvement in abilities in this area can be achieved through appropriate therapy. We know, for example, that ability in mathematics is greatly helped by actual handling and counting of objects, rather than simply dealing with numbers. Progress in early reading is strongly promoted by the writing of words and sentences.

Seeing and balance is important. If a child has poor gross motor coordination, he is unstable in space. When unstable in space, he encounters more difficulty in judging where things are in space.

The child needs to have experiences in developing eye-hand activities--going from gross motor activities, throwing and catching a ball, to the fine motor activity of seeing and being able to manipulate a pencil to write or a crayon to color within lines.

The child also needs experiences in coordinating what he hears with what he sees and feels. He needs experiences in judging distances, in seeing differences in size, color, weight, etc. A child also needs experiences in remembering what he has seen. Play provides the practice and the repetition which stimulates memory. Play also enables the development of concepts within the child's frame of reference.

Central processing has many elements. A child's play is his school up until he enters school. School readiness tests are tests of abilities which are themselves the result of a long series of abilities which the child needs to develop, many of which were begun in preschool play experiences.

To be most effective, testing in this area has to consider the quality of the input of each of the other perceptual systems in order to achieve best results. This input is integrated through the background of experience into the abilities to synthesize, categorize and to evaluate.

When, in a program of therapy, improvement in the performance of all three areas--sensory, motor and central processing--is achieved and the whole process of vision is operating well, many children are enabled to achieve in their classroom work at higher levels, some even rising from early failing grades to making the merit and honor rolls. A case in point was President Johnson's daughter, who was enabled to achieve much higher grades in college, following therapy, than she achieved in high school. It was doubtful, in fact, that she could have finished college without this treatment.

Just as in hearing and speech, providing a hearing aid, if needed, is often not enough for great improvement. In vision, also, providing glasses is often not enough. Improvement can be achieved through therapy to improve the functioning of the total process of vision with all areas acting efficiently together as a unit.

If a child exhibits symptoms of difficulty in these areas, it is important to seek out professionals in your community who examine and provide therapy for all three areas of vision: sensory, motor and central processing. Just to refer for an eye examination is not what is required. The examination and care must provide for all three areas of vision--sensory, motor and central processing.

All doctors in the field of vision care do not provide service for all three areas. Some doctors consider factors in the sensory area only. Other doctors consider factors in the motor mechanisms also. To test factors in the motor mechanisms, the eyes must be tested in their normal state. Tests in the motor mechanisms cannot be made if the doctor has used drops for testing in the sensory area. The drops are used to paralyze the focus mechanism while testing for refractive errors and, thus, focus ability cannot be tested as long as the drops are effectively paralyzing the muscles controlling focus.

A growing number of doctors are including central processing in their examinations and thus provide service for all three areas. It is important to know the service needed and where it is available in your community. If the parents take the child to a doctor who covers only the sensory area in the examination, then the child may not receive the services he needs, and both time in getting help to the child and financial resources are wasted.

IV.

VISION DEMANDS OF THE CLASSROOM

These are some of the important visual skills which are required for achievement in the normal classroom environment, all of them part of the total process of vision as discussed in the preceding sections of this manual:

a. To see clearly at distance and near.

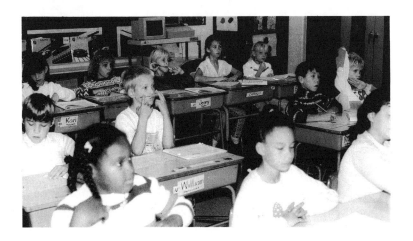

Children need to see clearly at all distances--chalkboard, desk and book--and in between distances. Children who do not see clearly at distance may see quite clearly at lesser distances, particularly desk and book distances. This occurs more often in the upper elementary grades as many become nearsighted.

b. To maintain binocular (two-eyed) fixation at either distance or near as needed.

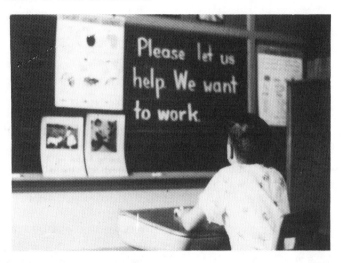

Children need to be able to maintain vision concentration easily at all distances. Several vision abilities in the motor area are involved. Maintaining vision concentration may be easier at board or at desk distances or may be difficult at all distances.

c. To change fixation easily from one place to another as in copying from a book or paper or from one part of a page to another.

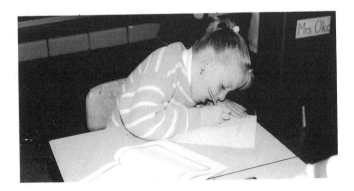

d. To change fixation from desk work to board work easily and back again for desk work.

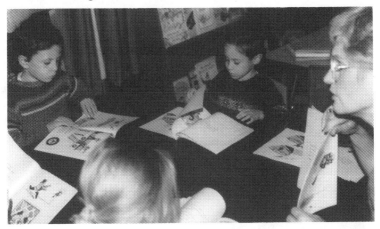

This is a learned activity, not congenital. In one study, 75% of kindergartners could not move fixation readily from one place to another. They need to be able to change fixation easily from one place to another and to keep their places in reading.

e. To follow across the page and from one line to the next line.

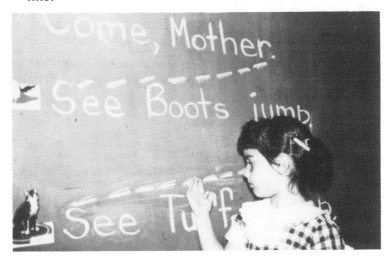

f. To maintain focus at far or near and to change focus easily.

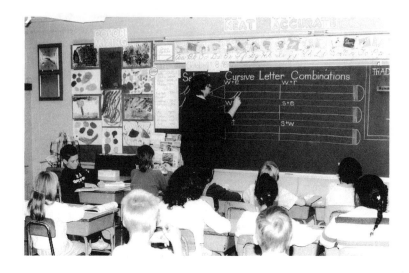

Children need to be able to maintain focus (for clear vision) at board and desk distances and to be able to change focus easily. Some children do not do this readily. The focus mechanism may not be functioning well so that focus itself is difficult or works slowly--causing the child to take more than the usual amount of time when changing focus from one distance to the other. Children need to be able to maintain single, clear vision at board and desk distances with ease. Some report doubling of words or blurring of words as they continue to work. These symptoms are very important.

g. To perceive likenesses and differences in form.

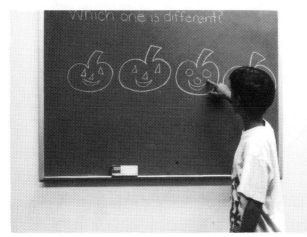

They need to be able to perceive likenesses and differences in form and size. The use of practice with geometric figures does not really contribute to the skill of word recognition, although this is a common practice. At the readiness stage, this is a common practice valuable for other reasons.

h. To perceive size and space relationships.

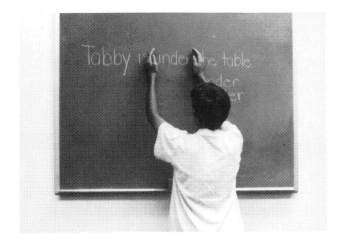

i. To perceive general configuration.

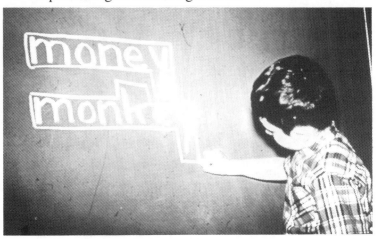

j. To have visual memory.

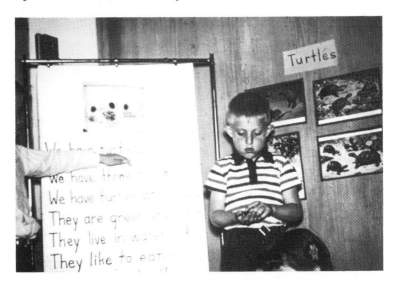

They need to develop visual memory. They need to learn to store visual images in memory and they need to be able to retrieve them.

k. To be able to visualize--to picture in their minds.
Children need to learn to visualize (picture in their minds). There is concern that when children watch television they do not gain experience in picturing in their minds the activity taking place--it is all on the screen. Nothing needs to be visualized. When children are read to, the picture of the activity is formed in their minds and becomes very much their own experience. This is why televised books or stories might not please everyone. Visualizations are personal and are an ability needed to aid comprehension.

l. To have good eye-hand coordination.

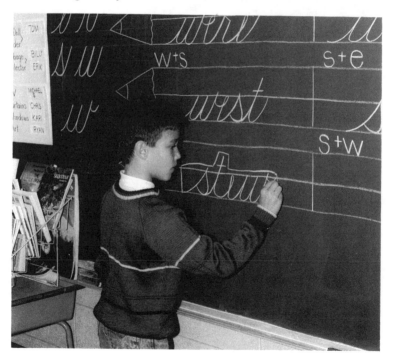

for writing skills

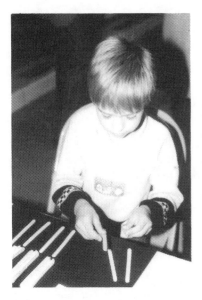
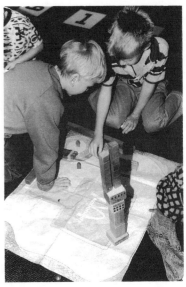

for manipulating things

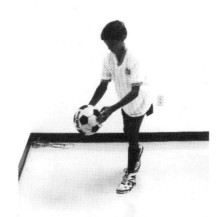

for sports

Children need to have good eye-hand coordination, not only for sports, but also for writing skills. Because of note taking in the upper grades and prolonged written examinations, it is important that children develop good writing skills early.

m. To be able to determine color.

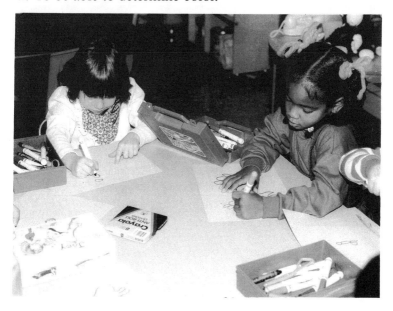

This is important especially in regard to having the child feel comfortable about school work. Although less than one percent of girls have difficulty, about eight percent of boys have difficulty perceiving colors as others perceive them. As adults they can tell about the difficulty they had in school because they were "color blind" and could not tell the difference between red and green and were thought not to be paying attention. Most color blind people are really color weak. They see colors but perceive them differently from normal people. Only a few perceive no color at all--seeing things in shades of gray. The teacher needs to know what the child can do.

We have up to this point reviewed the total process of vision as it operates when learning takes place by means of seeing, and have now reviewed important vision demands in the classroom. What does the teacher have available to understand each child and what can be done to help the child achieve in the classroom when learning takes place by means of seeing?

Areas of the Vision Process

Sensory	Motor			Central Processing
Refractive Error Visual Acuity Pathology	Eye Movement Efficiency	Focus & Focus Facility	Fusion & Ability to Maintain Fusion	Perceptual Abilities

V.

INFORMATION AVAILABLE TO CLASSROOM TEACHERS THROUGH SCHOOL SYSTEMS

Information through School Health Screening

Information from the school nurse will vary from one community to another. If there is screening of vision at all, the Snellen chart will probably be the instrument of choice.

The Snellen chart is used to determine whether or not the individual can see and is able to perceive detail that the average person can perceive at given distances. The term used for such testing is visual acuity testing. The average person has 20/20 visual acuity because he can perceive the certain sized letters shown on the Snellen at a distance of 20 feet. This 20- foot distance is the distance at which the Snellen test was devised. Such screening comes under Sensory (A) in the diagram of the total vision process.

Snellen testing provides information as to whether each separate eye sees clearly at 20 feet when it is tested alone. It tells us nothing about what the child actually sees when using both eyes in usual situations. In testing with both eyes seeing the target, one eye may see clearly while the other does not if each eye does not have the same refractive error. It also does not give information as to whether or not the child can see clearly at book and desk distances.

In testing the child who is nearsighted, differences in the optical power of each eye will show up in acuity testing with the Snellen chart when one eye perceives the detail of letters on one line and the other eye a different line.

In testing the farsighted child, each eye usually can achieve normal visual acuity when tested alone, but may not when both eyes are used at the same time if the refractive error is different for each eye. The input from each eye into the cortex should be equally clear for optimum visual performance.

School health screening usually reveals only one vision problem-- nearsightedness in one or both eyes. Unfortunately, nearsightedness is not related to school failure since most school work is at nearpoint. Nearsighted children do better in school than average children. Farsighted children who pass the Snellen may have real problems with book and desk tasks. Hence, screening by the Snellen does not yield the information that schools want to know.

Additional screening instruments to the Snellen chart often used are the Titmus and Keystone Telebinocular. The Titmus and the Telebinocular are essentially the same. They might look different, both in regard to the appearance of the instrument and the targets used with the instruments. However, they were designed by the same person who changed their appearance when he moved from one company to the other. They can screen for the same visual conditions.

These screening programs include tests in the motor mechanisms area. Therefore, they provide more information concerning the functioning of the total process of vision. They provide screening for factors affecting fusion at chalkboard and also at desk distance. Therefore, they are important tests to use.

None of the commercial screening programs available provides tests for eye movement control--pursuit and saccadic fixation, focus and focus facility, and central processing. The teacher will need to discuss with the person who does the special testing which areas are covered in the testing provided in this area.

In addition to the complexity of the vision process is the fact that seeing is personal; so much is brought to seeing from the reference point of the past experience of the perceiver and his present condition.

VI.

SYMPTOMS OF VISION DIFFICULTY AS DISPLAYED BY CHILDREN IN THE CLASSROOM

By learning how to observe the child, the informed class-room teacher has available very important information concerning the learning and performance abilities of each child. It is most important, therefore, that teachers become informed concerning symptoms of visual difficulty that children display by their behavior in the classroom. Teachers can become very effective screening instruments. They can observe the child day after day in dynamic situations. They have available to them symptoms of vision difficulty involving all areas, plus a knowledge of the factors of health, fatigue and emotion which affect visual performance, as well as other possible metacognitive factors, on a day to day basis. (Metacognitive: thought processes of the reader.)

Sensory

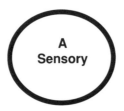

Vision problems in the sensory area of vision may lead to some of the following behaviors in the classroom:

a. A child straining or tilting the head to see when looking at board or chart work.

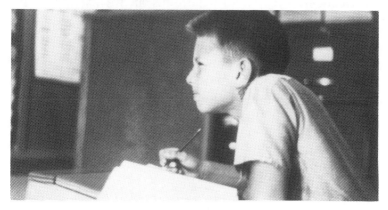

A child will tilt his head forward, or squint (almost close his eyes) in order to see more clearly. By so doing he allows light rays from the object fixated to enter his eye centrally--so the rays of light are affected least by the refractive error of the eye. This he has learned to do by trial and error as he tries to see more clearly. Such squinting may be temporarily effective, but it causes the activity to be stressful.

b. Signs of stress, rubbing eyes.

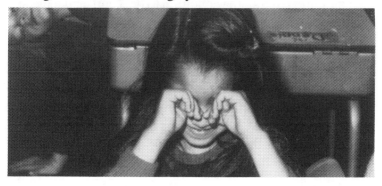

This may occur when viewing material on the chalkboard or watching a film or when reading is relatively prolonged. It shows up as a symptom under Sensory because of stress in trying to see more clearly.

c. Reddened eyes, encrusted eyelids, an eye that turns all the time.

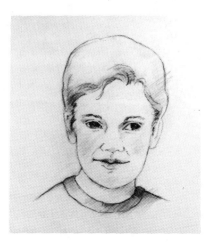

Here a drawing is used for obvious reasons. No child would wish to have his picture used showing such a problem. Since this problem is obvious, the parents and others are aware of the condition and aid is sought. If the eye turns all the time, then the child has a stable condition to deal with and it usually does not interfere with classroom learning. However, if an eye turns occasionally, then it is a real problem which will be discussed more fully under motor mechanisms.

d. Makes errors when copying from the board, but may not at book and desk distances. The child may make errors in copying from the board because of inability to see the work on the board clearly. To tell this, the teacher can simply see if the child does better if moved closer to the board. In nearsightedness, the child may have difficulty seeing board work but may see quite clearly at distance closer to him.

Motor Mechanisms

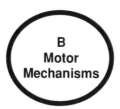

If poor performance is present in the motor mechanisms, children may display the following symptoms:

a. Avoidance of maintaining vision concentration, especially at book and desk distances.

1. By doing something else which you do not want him to do.

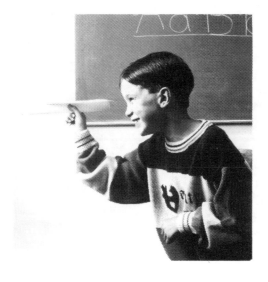

2. By daydreaming rather than working because it is too much effort to stay on task.

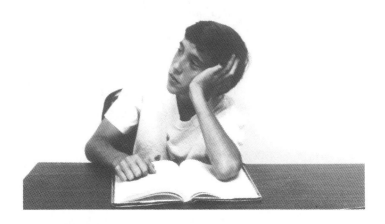

3. Staring off into space feeling unable to cope with the situation.

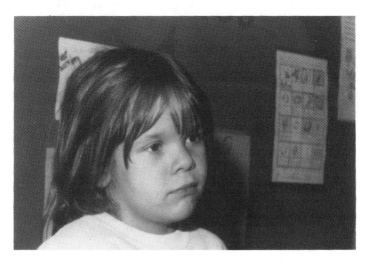

b. Avoiding the problem of having double vision by posture adjustments involving the use of only one eye.

    1. By turning head to use only one eye.

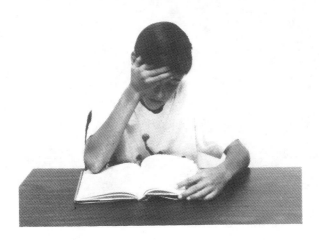

    2. By placing face close and tilting head, using only one eye.

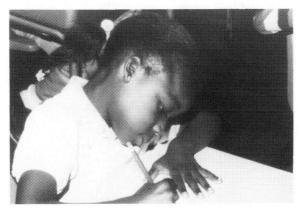

3. By covering one eye with hand while working.

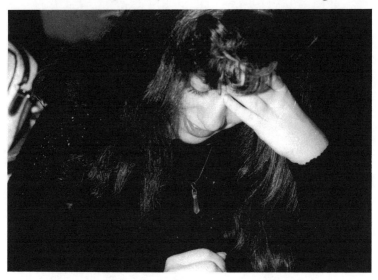

c. Struggling to maintain single binocular (both eyes) vision.

1. An eye that turns occasionally.

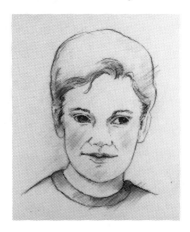

This is a very strong indication that the child is having

difficulty integrating the images from the two eyes into a single image.

d. Holding book closer to eyes or farther away than the distance from desk to face when it is measured by putting the closed fist against the cheek while resting the elbow on the desk. The child should hold his book or place his face as close to desk work as this distance to be in good physiological balance. Closer or farther away signals that there is some problem in the process in some area.
In noting this symptom, the teacher needs to be sure that the child's desk or table is not too close or farther away than normal. In this latter case the furniture would be causing a vision problem.

e. Persistent need to use finger to keep place in schoolwork. Frequently loses place in reading and desk work. Pointing to words is common at beginning reading levels because the motor mechanisms are weak. Only if it persists beyond primary age does it indicate a problem.

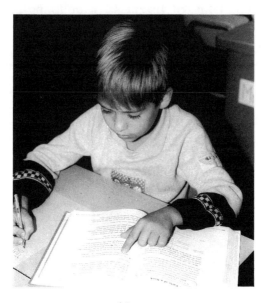

f. Also child may have difficulty locating items when moving eyes from chalkboard to desk work or to the book or in locating an item of present interest on a page.

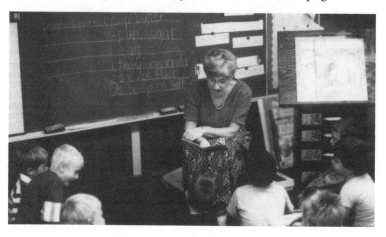

g. Some children indicate they have difficulty in the motor mechanisms by:
Watering eyes.
Reddened eyes after using eyes for reading and seat work.
Complaints of fuzziness or doubling print in book after reading a while.
Complaints of headaches as the day goes on and especially after using eyes for reading and seat work.
As reading and seat work are prolonged, the child becomes restless, irritable, or begins to make mistakes, reducing comprehension.

Central Processing

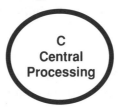

Indications of vision difficulty involving central processing are:

a. Needing to reinforce vision by saying and whispering the words.

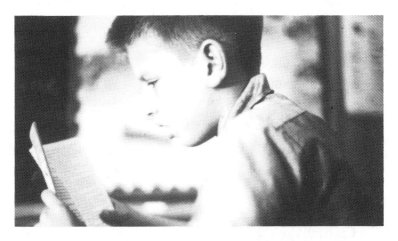

Moving lips and saying words aloud involving vocal cord movement. A student might say, "This is what I have to do to remember what I read," or the student can only understand material read aloud. Some pupils find it difficult to make the transition from oral to silent reading because of excessive emphasis upon oral in the early grades. Possibly the fact that most of their learning prior to entering school might have been by means of hearing, "Mama says," and not too much, "Look, and see for yourself."

b. Has to reread more than usual--so much effort goes into deciphering the words that comprehension of content is lost.

c. Poor comprehension--so much effort in perceiving and recognizing words that little attention is paid to what the words mean.

d. Poor visual memory--knows the word on one page, but not on the next, or knows the word one day, but not the next, showing difficulty in retrieving the word from memory. In severe cases, some children can spell a word, but cannot read it.

e. Unable to visualize--has not developed ability to picture in the mind the action taking place so that it has meaning.

f. Poor handwriting--can see but has difficulty reproducing what is seen. Writing is difficult, poorly formed and poorly spaced.

g. Can spell orally, but misspells when the word is written. Can spell for a spelling test but fails to recognize the word in reading. Can spell for a spelling test but not when asked to write the word in a sentence the same day or subsequently.

h. Makes more reversals than are expected for age or grade. Reversals are common in kindergarten. The proportion of reversals among first graders is about 40% and probably 10-20% in the second grade. For poor readers, the tendency persists indefinitely.

VII.

WHAT THE TEACHER CAN DO TO HELP THE CHILD AS LONG AS SYMPTOMS PERSIST

It is important that teachers be aware of symptoms of vision difficulty that children display in the classroom and continue to adjust their educational procedures and demands in terms of what the symptoms indicate as long as the symptoms persist. This is important because:

1. Considerable time may elapse between the time the child's difficulty is detected and when the parents seek appropriate aid for the child.
2. The parents do not understand the complexity of vision and simply seek aid in terms of what glasses can do to help the child see clearly for chalkboard distances.
3. It takes time with glasses and therapy to obtain the improvement needed in vision abilities. Some will require considerably more time than others.
4. Children with glasses may still have important abilities not functioning up to needed levels.

Symptoms are important because they provide important information concerning the child. We must ask "why" and seek to understand the "why" of deviant and unusual behavior rather than saying "that is the way some children do."

Sensory

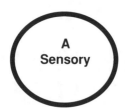

a. If the child has difficulty seeing board work and not with reading and seat work, be sure he sits as close to board and chart work as he needs to in order to see work presented there.

b. When possible provide a copy to use at book and desk distances if visual acuity seems adequate at these distances.

c. If trouble seeing clearly is present at all distances, then use bigger print, of good contrast, for seat work and reading. It is possible to purchase common school books and magazines printed in large size print. For example, Reader's Digest has such an edition.

d. All children showing symptoms of vision difficulty need to have material that is clear (size, contrast). The size of the print should be no smaller than that in text books for his grade level. The print in some workbooks is entirely too small. Small print in poorly reproduced materials presents an extra problem for children struggling to learn through means of a vision process which is not functioning efficiently.

Studies in optimum print size for various grade levels have recommended the following:

Grade 1	14-18 point type
Grades 2-3	14-16 point type
Grade 4	12 point type
Grades 5-8	10-12 point type

18 point type   Jane saw Tom.

16 point type   Jane saw Tom.

14 point type   Jane saw Tom.

12 point type   Jane saw Tom.

10 point type   Jane saw Tom.

These print sizes are reproduced here as a guide. We have seen school papers which were poorly reproduced (print not clear) and material printed in 10 point type given as an exercise at the second grade level. The smaller the print the greater the demand on focus. The greater the demand on focus the more stress there may be encountered in easily maintaining clear vision at book and desk distances. Some children even report they encounter seeing two sets of words rather than just one or have temporary blurring of work.

If the child is struggling to learn and shows these symptoms of vision difficulty, the resourceful teacher can help by not using materials which are in small print and poorly reproduced. Some copying machines will enlarge materials as they copy them.

Motor Mechanisms

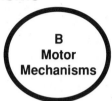

a. If child shows more symptoms of difficulty at book and desk distances than for board and chart distances, present as much of the work at board and chart distances as possible.

b. Give child time when possible to locate his place in board work and book and seat work. Help him find it by pointing to it or underlining or using a marker.

c. For seat work, permit the child to use a marker or his finger to aid him in keeping his place. Some children even benefit by having most of the page, except what is being considered, covered. Adjustments may vary from all being covered except the material to which the child is to attend, to merely using the finger to keep the place or using a marker to stay on line. Using a finger or marker is a symptom that the eye-aiming mechanism is not functioning as well as needed. Here, we allow the child to use these crutches until they are no longer needed. He needs the crutches to have some chance of achieving. If he is having therapy and is in a training program, the specialist doing the training should inform the teacher when the child should be encouraged to cease using a crutch.

d. If when the child is required to maintain vision concentration at book and desk distances for prolonged periods, there is stress evidenced by:

1. Being restless or showing difficulty keeping on task.
2. Tilting head to one side, covering one eye, placing face close to desk so as to use one eye only.
3. Performing less well the longer the child works.
4. Complaints of headaches, rubbing eyes, eyes becoming watery, saying print jumps around or becomes fuzzy.

Give the child shorter assignments, allowing frequent breaks from desk distance activities by changing what you ask the child to do.

e. If there are indications the child can learn more easily by means of hearing, allow the child opportunities to reinforce vision by means of hearing and to indicate what he has learned by oral testing until his ability to learn by means of seeing can be improved through appropriate therapy.

f. If a child is wearing glasses that cause one eye to look smaller than the other eye, this child may need to be a head turner, moving his head to make fixations on words as he moves along a line of print. When the lens for one eye differs significantly from that of the other, it creates a problem. To cope with it, the child has to move his head rather than his eyes to keep from seeing double. The child should be allowed to move his head rather than his eyes under such circumstances. The doctor providing therapy should be consulted as to the best way to handle this problem.

A correction for farsightedness also magnifies what is looked at. A correction for nearsightedness minifies. At the same time, when looking through other than the center of the lens, a lens can also, according to the power of the lens, have a prismatic effect. A prism causes an object to be perceived at a different place than it actually is, according to the strength of the prism.

The magnification factor puts a stress on fusion because of size differences. If the difference in perceived sizes becomes too great, it is difficult to fuse the two images. The prismatic factor puts a stress on fusion because one eye perceives what is looked at to be in one place, the other perceives it at a slightly different place. If the difference in perceived placement is too great, then fusion becomes difficult or impossible. By turning the head, so as to be always looking through the center of the lenses of his glasses, the child can avoid the prismatic effect of the lenses he must wear to see clearly with each eye.

Contact lenses, because each fits on the surface of its eye, do not produce as much difference in size, and produce no prismatic effect at all as long as each lens remains centered on the eye. Hence, they do not produce this problem for children or adults.

Central Processing

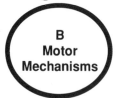

a. Allow the primary child to use a marker or finger to keep his place in school--his finger reinforcing vision. Some children need this because of figure-ground difficulty. They need help in maintaining their attention on a particular word, pulling it out from the words around it.

b. For writing skills:
   1. Be sure child holds pencil properly and that paper is

parallel to his writing hand. To hold the pencil properly, the pencil should be held with the third finger underneath the pencil, the index finger on top of the pencil and the thumb at the side of the pencil. The fourth and little fingers rest on the desk and are not involved in holding and manipulating the pencil except to cushion the hand on the desk. A rubber band placed at least one inch from the point of the writing instrument helps children assume proper holding position. The child is taught to keep his fingers on or above the rubber band. Thus he can see what he writes and there is no need for twisting the hand as so many do. Little plastic pieces that slip over the pencil (available through school supply stores) help the child learn to use the correct fingers and to hold the pencil at the correct distance from the point of the pencil.

Paper position is important in developing good writing ability. In other words, for the right-handed child the upper right hand corner of the page should be above and to the right of his writing hand. The paper is tilted in this fashion. For the left- handed child, the paper is tilted so that the upper left corner is above and to the left of his writing hand. This enables the left-handed child to have the same slant in his writing as do others.

It is important to watch left-handed children to be sure their paper is positioned for left-handed writing. When they start learning to write, it is important also to watch left-handed children as they learn to write from left to right. It is thought the natural movement is away from the midline of the body. This would make it more natural for a left-handed child to write from right to left. Therefore, left-handed children need to be watched carefully as they learn to write from left to right.

2. Use lined paper, heavily lined if need be, to call attention to space restrictions. Some letters are one space, others two spaces, and one lower case letter in cursive occupies three spaces: .

   c. Allow the child to whisper to himself or read aloud so that the auditory process can reinforce the vision process (if this proves helpful). However, eventually the reader must become a silent reader. Practicing whispering, or reading aloud delays this maturation. It should not be permitted above primary grades. A pencil held crosswise in the mouth or something to chew tends to discourage whispering.

   d. If he learns easily by hearing and earphones are available, let the child use them--hearing the words while seeing them. But most children cannot keep their places while following the tapes produced by adult readers. If a portion of the tape is heard prior to attempting to read the material, the child's performance may be helped.

   e. In spelling, especially, it has been found to be helpful to have the child reinforce vision by saying and writing the material considered, involving other sensory modalities in a meaningful way. Have the child say the letters while writing them: saying the word, then writing the word-- saying, hearing and seeing the letters in the word while writing them. Sometimes it is helpful to have the child close his eyes and then write the word in the air with the finger while the eyes are closed-- visualizing the word as written. Also, it has proven helpful to have child say words in syllables and in slow motion so as to obtain a road map of sounds in the word. Ask the child to listen to the sounds as heard in the word and then account for what is heard by using the letters which make the sounds heard. Because of all the irregular words in our language, there are many words which cannot be spelled easily by means of what is heard.

Exercises which help the child learn to perceive details, differences in detail of letters in words, can be helpful, as well as exercises to help develop visual memory. There are many materials available to help develop these abilities.

VIII.

SUMMARY OF VISION AS IT OPERATES FOR LEARNING

Vision, as it operates for learning, for many reasons cannot be illustrated by means of a camera, even if we considered two cameras, one for each eye. Many parts of the total system would not be accounted for. Vision is more adequately explained in terms of computers rather than a simple camera.

Vision needs to be understood as a complex process that what is seen (perceived) is personal, depending greatly on the functioning of the Sensory--seeing clearly; Motor--combining easily the two inputs, one from each eye, keeping the single image obtained in clear focus at all distances; and Central Processing-- opportunities to develop needed abilities resulting from combining vision with the input from the other sensory systems in order to clothe the input with meaning, with all three systems acting together as a unit.

Teachers can help:
1. By gaining some perspective on the complexity of vision as a total process.
2. By considering the many vision demands of the classroom.
3. By becoming informed and thus aware of the symptoms of vision difficulty children display in their classroom behavior.
4. By searching out professional help for the children needing it.
5. By adjusting teaching methods in light of the abilities a child has or does not have as long as symptoms of

difficulty persist.

Teachers may thus play a very important role in a child's success. In this we move away from labeling a child in terms of his disabilities, adjusting our methods and expectations accordingly to helping the child develop needed abilities and thus being able to achieve in terms of his true potential.

APPENDIX

Symptoms of Vision Difficulty As Displayed in the Classroom

Name _____

Sensory

Straining or tilting head to see   _____

Signs of stress   _____

    eyes water   _____

    rubbing eyes   _____

Reddened eyes, encrusted eyelids,
    an eye that turns   _____

Makes errors when copying from the
    board, but not at book and desk distances   _____

Motor Mechanisms

Avoidance of maintaining vision concentration,
    especially at book and desk distances   _____

    by doing something else which you
        do not want him to do   _____

    by daydreaming rather than working--
        too much effort to stay on task   _____

Staring off in space,
    feeling unable to cope with task   _____

Avoiding the problem of having double
    vision by posture adjustments involving
    the use of one eye   _____

    by turning head to use only one eye   _____

    by placing head close and tilting head   _____

    by covering one eye with hand while working   _____

Struggling to maintain single, binocular (both eyes) vision _____
    an eye that turns (in or out) occasionally _____
    persistent need to use finger to keep
        place in schoolwork _____
    loses place frequently in reading and desk work _____
    has difficulty locating items when moving eyes from
        chalkboard to desk work or to the book _____
    difficulty locating an item of present interest
        on a page _____
    watering eyes _____
    reddened eyes _____
    complaints of headaches _____
    as reading and seat work are prolonged,
        becomes restless _____

Central Processing

needs to reinforce vision by saying and
    whispering the words _____
has to reread _____
poor comprehension _____
poor visual memory _____
unable to visualize _____
poor handwriting _____
can spell orally but misspells when written _____
makes more reversals than are expected for age or grade _____

Optimum Working Distance for Book and Desk work to be in Physiological Balance

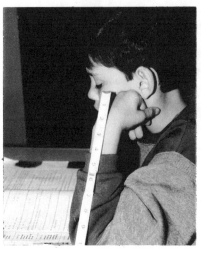

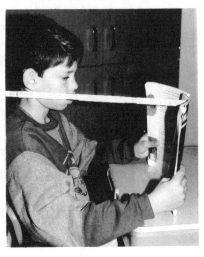

Measuring the distance from desk to face by putting the closed fist against the cheek while resting the elbow on the desk.

Holding the book at this optimum distance.

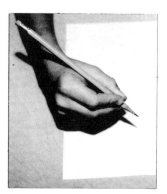

Holding Pencil Correctly

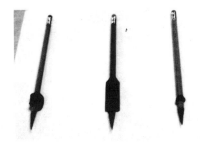

Aids to Learning to Hold Pencil Correctly

ABOUT THE AUTHORS

George D. Spache, Ph.D.

After receiving his B.A. degree from New York University Dr. Spache spent six years as an elementary school teacher. He then pursued graduate work and in 1938 received his Ph.D. from N.Y.U. He spent 14 years as a school psychologist in public and private schools and as a consulting psychologist in industry. He also taught at New York and Rutgers Universities.

In 1949 he founded the Reading Laboratory and Clinic at Florida University and served as its head for two decades. During this period he was also a visiting professor at seven different American universities as well as those of Johannesburg, South Africa, Dalhousie of Halifax, Nova Scotia, and Massey University of New Zealand.

With Dr. Evelyn Spache, he directed International Institutes for American teachers for five consecutive years in Leysin, Switzerland, Bangkok, Thailand, and the American Virgin Islands. They also participated in reading conferences in several European countries, Hong Kong and Australia. Dr. Spache has presented at reading and optometric conferences in 40 states and Canada.

Among his awards are the Apollo Award of the American Optometric Association, the Citation of Merit of the International Reading Association, the Layman's Award of the Florida Optometric Association, Fellow of the American Academy of Optometry and Diplomate of the American Psychological Association. He has published more than 100 articles and 50 books and tests including: the "Binocular Reading Test," a measure of the functioning of children's vision in the act of reading; the "Diagnostic Reading Scales," a reading test series; and "Children's Vision," a slide presentation created in collaboration with his fellow author, Lois B. Bing, A.B., O.D.

Lillian R. Hinds, Ph.D

D r. Hinds received her B.A. in 1941 and M.A. in 1951 from Western Reserve and her Ph.D. in 1966 from Case Western Reserve. She has taught at the Case Western Reserve University Reading Clinic, served as Language Arts Supervisor and Director of Vision Screening for the Euclid, Ohio public schools where she collaborated with Dr. Lois Bing to develop a vision screening program. She was a professor at Cleveland State University where she earned the Mitau Award for innovative programs awarded by the American Association of State Universities and Colleges and in 1988 she received the Ohio Optometric Association's Distinguished Service Award.

Dr. Hinds served as president of the Ohio Reading Council and of the Arizona Reading Council of the International Reading Association.

A Professor Emerita from Cleveland State University, Dr. Hinds continues as editor of the *Journal of Clinical Reading: Research and Programs,* a publication of the Clinical Division, College Reading Association. She is a former editor of *Education Horizons* for Pi Lambda Theta, an honorary educational society.

At the invitation of the village of Manual Diegiez, Jalisco, Mexico, Dr. Hinds taught in the village and ranch schools, providing in-service demonstrations for their professional staff.

Her published works include "A Research Trilogy: American and Mexican Vision Studies." These studies include the results of vision research done in the Euclid, Ohio public schools, in the Arizona Reading Improvement School, and in Manual Diegiez, Mexico. Other publications are "The Short Test of Representational Levels: A Language Model and Personalized Management Activities"; "The Spelling Patterns Test"; "Visual Motor Perceptual Training Program"; "A Decade of Innovative Approaches to Beginning Reading: Studies in the Use of Color"; "Success in Reading,"a handbook for tutors for Developing Ohio Citizens (DOC) (juvenile delinquency); "Adventures in Seeing"; and "Readiness and Success in Reading."

Lois B. Bing, A.B., O.D.

After receiving her A.B. and teaching credential in 1931 from the College of Wooster, Wooster, Ohio, Dr. Bing earned her optometry degree in 1948 from the College of Optometry at Ohio State University. She continued her interest in education through graduate studies at Ohio State, Pittsburgh and Case Western Reserve Universities. She has participated in one cross-sectional study of the relationship of vision and reading (grades two, four, six, eight) and two six-year longitudinal studies. In addition, she has participated in informal studies of the relationship of strabismus and reading achievement and vision and school readiness. In collaboration with Dr. Lillian R. Hinds, she devised the vision screening program for the Euclid, Ohio, schools and served as their vision consultant for many years. She collaborated with Dr. George D. Spache in producing a slide presentation on "Vision and School Success."

Dr. Bing chaired the Visual Problems of Children and Youth Committee of the American Optometric Association for a period of 12 years from 1951-1963. During that time she prepared the American Optometric Association's report to the 1960 White Conference on Children and Youth. She has been a speaker for education and optometric audiences throughout the United States.

Dr. Bing has written articles on vision and reading for *The Reading Teacher, The Journal of Learning Disabilities* and *Clinical Reading*, as well as various optometric publications. In recognition of her work on vision and reading Dr. Bing was presented the Apollo Award for distinguished service by the American Optometric Association, made an Honorary Life Member of the American Academy of Optometry and an Honorary Life Member of the Ohio Council of the International Reading Association and the Ohio School Psychologists Association, as well as Delta State Chapter of Delta Kappa Gamma, International. She received a special commendation from the College of Optometry at Ohio State University for "exceptional service to our profession in the area of children's vision and learning disorders and for her continuing dedication to the visual well-being of humanity."

Since 1951, Dr. Bing has chaired the School Vision Forum and Reading Conference which presents nationally prominent speakers in the fields of education, psychology and optometry.